Foreword

National audits give the opportunity for practitioners to compare their practice with others throughout the country. They are, therefore, potentially powerful tools for change. However, some national audits are more successful than others and some clinicians make better use of national audits than do others.

Taking part in a national audit carries with it a commitment to change practice if, as a result, that practice is found to be sub-optimal. This commitment can be time-consuming and should not be underestimated. It is therefore important for clinicians to be able to judge whether it is worth participating in a national audit, for example on the grounds of their involvement with the topic to be audited, the importance of that topic to patient care, and the quality of the audit itself.

This book is designed to help clinicians and managers decide whether they should take part in national audit, and how to make lasting improvements in practice as a result of their participation. Written by two people with experience of running national audits, this book is a very practical guide to using such audits to improve practice and is strongly commended to you.

November 2000   PROFESSOR SIR GEORGE ALBERTI
                                   President, Royal College of Physicians

The Clinical Effectiveness and Evaluation Unit (CEEU) of the Royal College of Physicians

The Clinical Effectiveness and Evaluation Unit of the Royal College of Physicians concentrates on those issues that are at the centre of the national healthcare agenda, eg the National Service Frameworks in Cardiology, Care of Older People and Diabetes, and the Calman-Hine Cancer Framework, as a continuous programme of work rather than multiple one-off projects. Associate Directors, who are active clinicians in their field, lead the relevant programmes in conjunction with the Director. CEEU has expertise in the development of guidelines, the organising and reporting of multi-centre comparative audit to encourage guideline implementation, and studies on how the outcome of care can be measured reliably. All our work is collaborative with relevant specialist societies, patient groups and health service bodies such as the National Service Frameworks, National Institute for Clinical Excellence (NICE) and, in future, the Centre for Health Improvement (CHI). CEEU is self-financing with funding coming from government, charities and other organisations.

Contents

Introduction

The Royal Colleges and professional bodies have been organising national clinical audits for some years. They range from the national confidential enquiries – with their focus on significant events such as the death of a patient – to audits of specific conditions or procedures. Although the results of the national confidential enquiries are kept confidential, the organisers of national clinical audits are increasingly encouraging clinical teams to share their results with others. This allows clinical teams to learn from each other and compare themselves more openly with similar teams in other parts of the country.

National clinical audits can be powerful tools for improving practice across the whole country. They are becoming much more fashionable, and up to about twenty national clinical audits may be in operation at any one time. However, they should not be undertaken lightly or they will end up as little more than data collection exercises.

This booklet looks at how local clinical teams can get the most out of participating in a national clinical audit. It will take you through deciding whether your team should participate, establishing a local project team, what the results of the audit mean for you, deciding whether and what you need to change, and how to make the change process work.

Flow charts are included for each stage of the audit denoting the questions that need to be asked and answered, and the issues to be addressed or acted on.

Flow chart to show the process of participating in a national clinical audit from deciding to take part to improving practice.

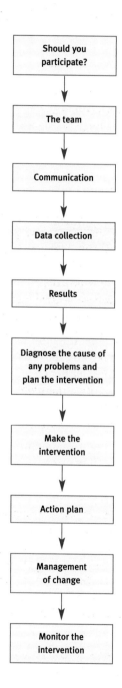

1 National clinical audits: should you participate?

Participating in a national clinical audit will commit you and your colleagues to a lot of work. Before you commit to taking part in a national clinical audit, there are a few questions that you need to ask yourself and the organisers:

How committed are you to this topic?

Ideally, the topic of the audit should be an area of practice that is both important and one with a wide variation in practice. If you and your team do not think the topic is important, it is unlikely that you will want to spend a lot of time on the audit. If there is little variation in practice or little room for improvement, the effort required in conducting the audit may be misplaced. Commitment to the audit should include a commitment to change practice if the results show a need for improvement. It will also usually include a commitment to conduct a re-audit at a later stage.

Ask yourself:
► Is the topic of the audit a priority either nationally or locally?
► Do you find it interesting enough to take part?
► Are you willing to make a commitment to change practice if necessary?

Who is organising the audit?

The organisers of the audit should be a credible group, with expertise in the area being audited and the organisational skills to be able to manage a large project. This will usually mean an academic institution, a Royal College or professional body. The funding for the project should also come from a credible institution: for example, the Department of Health has funded several national clinical audits. Funding from sources such as the pharmaceutical industry could lead to questions of bias in the design or organisation of the audit.

Most national clinical audits will be run by a collaboration of two or more bodies. These will usually represent all the professions and specialties involved in the area being audited. If there are any obvious omissions you should question whether this would bias the audit: for example, an audit involving only medical Royal Colleges will concentrate on medical interventions while potentially missing inputs by nursing and other professions.

Ask yourself:
- ▶ Is the organising group credible?
- ▶ Are all the relevant professions and specialties represented?

On what evidence is the audit based?

Any audit must have a standard, or series of standards, to audit against. The standards for a national clinical audit must be explicit and it should be clear that the standards are derived from good research evidence. A good source of national standards is clinical guidelines which, by their construction, lend themselves to audit:

They are systematically developed statements to assist practitioner and patient decisions about appropriate healthcare for specific clinical circumstances.[1]

If a national clinical audit is not based on clinical guidelines, the research on which it is based should be high quality and generally accepted as good practice.

Ask yourself:
- ▶ Is the audit based on a clinical guideline or other high quality research evidence?

Is the methodology sound?

The methodology used in the audit should relate to the topic, particularly to the standards being audited against, and be sufficiently robust to answer the questions posed in the audit (Box 1). Detailed methodologies will often not be available when participants are being recruited, but you should ensure that you are happy with the methods being employed before finally agreeing to take part.

It is becoming more common for organisers of national clinical audits to start the process with a draft methodology that is then refined after consulting with the potential participants. This may present you with the opportunity to take part in piloting the audit. The benefits in being a pilot site is that it provides a chance to test out the audit and iron out any problems before collecting the main data.

Box 1

Points to consider when deciding on the appropriateness of the methodology include:[2]

▶ *Relationship between data collected and audit objectives*: the data collected should relate directly to the audit objectives and standards.
▶ *Sample size*: this should be adequate to give confidence in the accuracy of the results.
▶ *Inclusion/exclusion criteria*: the types of cases, episodes or occurrences and how they are selected should be clearly defined and relate to the audit objectives and standards.
▶ *Evidence and good practice*: the audit design should reflect up-to-date sound evidence of good practice. If research evidence is not available, it should reflect national consensus on good practice.
▶ *Use of valid tools*: any tools used in data collection (eg forms, surveys, etc) should have been properly validated before use.
▶ *Ethics*: the collection and use of data should meet accepted ethical principles. (*Note*: this does not mean that participation will necessarily require local research ethics committee approval.)
▶ *Confidentiality*: audit data should be collected, handled and presented in a manner consistent with Caldicott principles.[3]

You can expect to have an outline of the methodology, but many of the details will be finalised following the initial meetings with participants. Although this can seem frustrating, it is actually a good feature because the participants can influence the practicalities of the audit. There is a growing acceptance among those running national clinical audits that the participants have a role in refining the audit – and many will allow a degree of local variation.

Ask yourself:
▶ Is the methodology sound, relevant and robust?
▶ Can you have a say in the detail of the audit?
▶ Is the audit being piloted; if so, how (eg how many centres are piloting and over what period)?

What data are to be collected and by whom?

The organisers of the audit may not be able to tell you exactly what data will be collected until after the audit has been refined by the participants (see above). However, they should be able to tell you the amount of data that should be collected and whether local staff or the national clinical audit team will collect it.

You will need to assess whether the amount of data is reasonable in terms both of achieving the aims of the audit and of workload. It is also worth thinking about whether the data are quantitative, qualitative or a mix of both. Quantitative data identify the extent of the problem, whereas qualitative data give clues about the causes of a problem. The qualitative data may also reveal the strengths and weaknesses of a service or give people's perceptions and experiences of the service. An audit that provides a mixture of quantitative and qualitative data is likely to be most helpful.

The organisers of the audit should have thought about how they will check the reliability of the data, especially if the data will be collected by a number of different people in different sites. This quality assurance is important to ensure that true comparisons can be made.

Ask yourself:
- ▶ Is the amount of data to be collected reasonable and will it help you identify both the extent and the cause of any problems?
- ▶ Are there reliability checks on the data to take account of different data collectors?

How useful will the results be?

The big strength of national clinical audits is that they allow comparison between different groups or individuals, usually in the form of a comparison between your results and the pooled national data. Some national clinical audits go further, facilitating contact between similar sites, or feeding back the lessons learnt by other sites to encourage learning from each other. The comparative data should allow you to compare yourselves against similar sites with a similar case mix. This is important because it might be unreasonable to compare, for example, a tertiary referral centre with a district general hospital.

The results should be returned to you within a relatively short time after the data collection. You should ask how long it will be before your results are returned to you. If there is a long delay they will be less relevant when they arrive. In some national clinical audits you will do all the data collection and have the opportunity to review your own performance before the national results are available. This will allow you to form your own opinions about the results before comparing them with other units.

Ask the questions:
- ▶ How long will it take before your results are returned?
- ▶ Will you have access to your own results before the national results are available?
- ▶ Do the organisers encourage contact between different sites to allow joint learning?
- ▶ Will case mix be taken account of in the analysis?

Who do you need in your local project team?

Healthcare is increasingly delivered by teams of healthcare professionals working together. Improvements in healthcare will similarly depend on teams of people working together. If you want to use the results of a national clinical audit to improve the performance of your team, you will need to involve all the members of the team from the very beginning. This may well include the management of the trust/primary care group, etc.

Many national clinical audits give guidance about who to involve in the local project team. You should establish whether the organisers of the audit are issuing guidance and whether there needs to be any patient or carer involvement. If patient or carer involvement is recommended, the organisers should be able to advise on how to go about this.

Ask yourself:
- ▶ Is it clear who needs to be involved in the local project team?

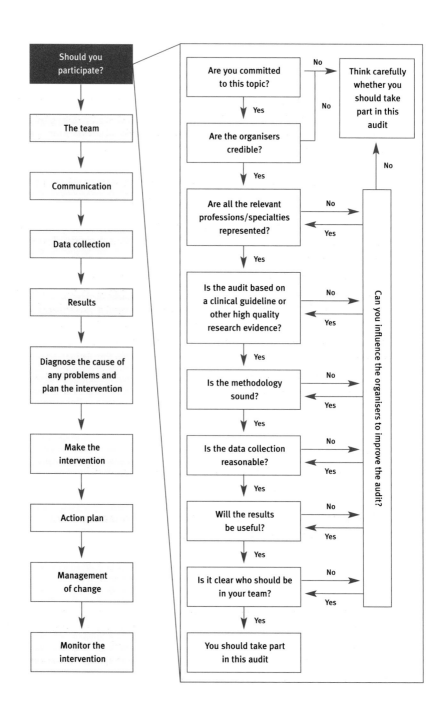

2 The team

In order to facilitate change, all relevant specialties need to agree that a change in practice is necessary, and that support for implementation initiatives will be forthcoming from essential stakeholders, management and clinical staff. The most important prerequisite for a successful team is a commitment to working together towards a shared goal. Physically signing an agreement to take part and, if necessary, to implement change can improve people's personal commitment to a project.

Experience from Action on Clinical Effectiveness and Promoting Action on Clinical Effectiveness[4] has shown that effective teams combining people from clinical and management backgrounds and skills encourage action and result in improvement in practice. It is critical that the right people are on the team to ensure a successful improvement. Teams will vary in both size and composition, and each group needs to build a team that will suit its own local needs. In some situations there may be a natural inclination to concentrate on clinicians to lead the team and undertake the work. This may not be wholly appropriate, however, since different individuals may possess skills that make them better equipped for the task in hand.

Planning initiatives to improve a healthcare system will require answers to the following questions:
▶ What is the aim of the project?
▶ What processes will be affected by the improvement?
▶ Who needs to be involved?

When forming a team, there needs to be a sound management approach with clear definition of the following:

Who will lead the work?

It is imperative that the 'right' person is identified to lead the work since the management of change is a complex and lengthy process. This individual needs to be able to influence others, and to have a level of authority or influence in all areas affected by change. There may be resource implications when such initiatives are instituted which will necessitate cross-departmental and organisational discussions that can be facilitated by opinion leaders or high status individuals.

Who will undertake day-to-day co-ordination?

An individual – usually someone different to the project leader – needs to take responsibility for the day-to-day management of the project: ideally somebody who works routinely in the area being tackled and who therefore has a thorough understanding of the process. This will lend credibility to the change being instituted and may be accepted with greater ease within the group. Additionally, this individual should have an understanding of the various effects of the planned changes on the process, and both a desire and the ability to drive the project on a daily basis.

Who will do the work?

An accurate assessment of the resources required in terms of manpower, time and materials is essential to ensure change is managed successfully. The project team may have all the necessary skills and abilities within it to do this, but may need support from management, the information technology department or clinical audit department.

Teams should be aware of the potential workload involved before agreeing to take part in the audit. Without this commitment at the start they will be unlikely to follow through on time-consuming elements of either the audit or the change.

Who should make up the team?

This will depend upon the nature of the project. Some projects do not stipulate the composition of the team, but a general rule would be that every profession involved in the delivery of care to the patient group being audited should be represented on the team. Other expertise, such as audit and management expertise, may be needed in order successfully to run the audit or to implement change. It is important that all individuals within the team have definite roles of which they are aware, so that they are able to relate to one another to produce a cohesive working group and so that their skills are used to maximal benefit. Some changes may require input from the management of the trust or practice, or may have resource implications. It is helpful to have gained the commitment of senior management to the project from the start, which may mean including a manager in the project team.

Within this handbook there is guidance on developing action plans, in which it is imperative that all members of the team are involved. This will ensure sharing of the workload, as well as a commitment to succeed since individuals will undertake discrete activities that will lead to overall improvement.

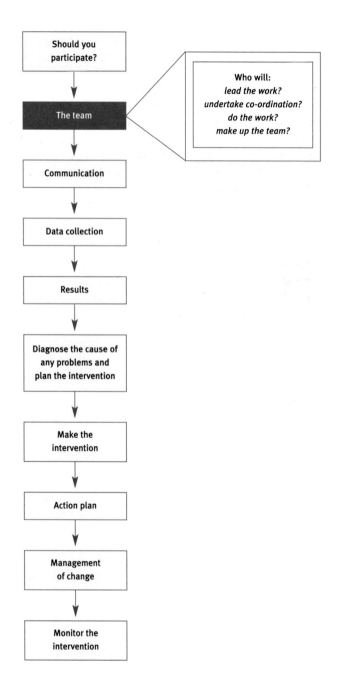

3 Communication

Communication is the key to success! It helps to ensure the wide involvement of people and encourages individuals to become part of the change process. Communication not only includes the dissemination of information and taking part in discussion – members of the team also need to listen to each other and to value individual contributions. This will encourage an atmosphere of team working and the sharing of knowledge, skills and expertise.

Methods of communication

Communication needs to be tailored to achieve the desired benefit. A variety of methods can – and should – be used (Box 2). It is vital that all participants are able to express their opinions in a non-threatening environment conducive to team work.

Box 2

Examples of communication methods:

Verbal

▶ Meetings of the whole project team
▶ Meetings of the core members of the team to deal with an aspect of the project
▶ One-to-one communication between members of the team
▶ Updates from the project team in other meetings to keep non-participants informed (eg departmental and board meetings)

Written

▶ Minutes of meetings of the project team or subgroups (these can be circulated to all members of the project team and to other interested groups)
▶ Newsletters from the project team
▶ Articles in trust newsletters, etc

Within the team

Team members should meet regularly to report progress and to discuss solutions to potential problems that may have been encountered. This will engender co-operation between team members and a sense of individual responsibility while working towards a collective goal. These teams will usually be multiprofessional, reflecting the healthcare approach used in most organisations. Such teams have a wealth of knowledge and skills of which it is important to make full use. When it comes to devising and monitoring your action plan for change (details are provided later in this handbook) all members within the team should contribute and, most importantly, be listened to by their colleagues on the team.

Within the healthcare organisation

Change does not occur in a vacuum, so a change in practice in one area may result in knock-on effects for other processes. For this reason, informing related groups within the healthcare organisation helps to ensure support of activities. Moreover, by involving related groups there may be increased commitment for the implementation of change as this can be considered an integral part of an overall strategy to improve health for the local population. In such cases, it may be appropriate for different members of the team to convey the messages to the different networks within an organisation (eg a pharmacist on the team may be the best person to feed back activities to the pharmacy department).

Management

The team must report at regular intervals to management within the healthcare organisation to show the benefit of the activity and the resultant health outcomes. This may provide an opportunity for additional resources to be made available if necessary. Management endorsement will also lend credibility to the change in activities, which may then stand a better chance of being accepted and implemented into clinical practice.

External to the healthcare organisation

When practice is changed, this will invariably reverberate through to other clinical and non-clinical settings not directly related to the organisation. It is valuable to communicate the successes and barriers encountered by the team in case groups in other sectors want to undertake similar activities. Health authorities and primary care groups will have a particular interest in any improvements made because of the audit. Patient groups and community health councils may also wish to know.

Communication across the primary/secondary care interface is encouraged with involvement of primary care groups and health authorities. This will help to ensure that there is little disparity in practice between the different sectors of patient care.

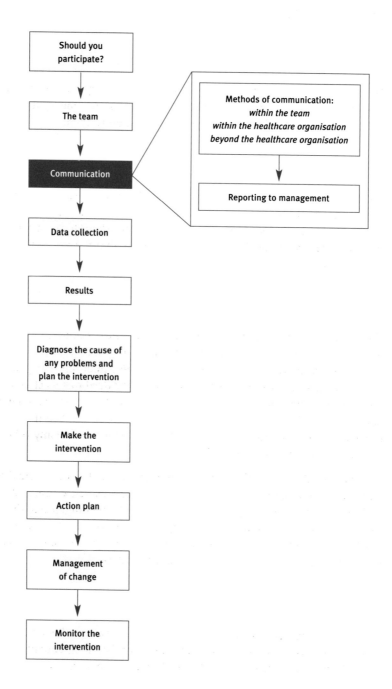

4 Data collection

Organisers of national audits take one of two broad approaches to data collection. They will either collect the data themselves using their own staff, or ask you to collect the data for transmission to them.

External data collection

If they are collecting the data for you, you will need to arrange for them to have access to the data they need. This may mean that you will have to arrange for a member of your staff to introduce them to ward staff or medical record staff, etc. You will have to ensure that the external data collectors follow Caldicott principles.[3]

Internal data collection

If the data collection will be your responsibility, there should be guidance from the organisers about what data should be collected and how to select the right patients for the audit. It is important that your data collectors understand exactly what data they need to collect and where those data can be found. Many national audits require looking in patients' notes for information. The people selected to perform the task of data collection should be familiar with patients' notes and any other sources of information used in the audit.

Many national audits include training sessions for staff undertaking the audit. The training may be aimed at both the local leaders of the audit and the data collectors. If possible, the people who will undertake the data collection should attend the training meeting. Where this is not possible, the person attending should take detailed notes about the data collection and be prepared to advise the data collectors.

Piloting the data collection

It is advisable to pilot the data collection on a few patients before the main audit; this is especially important for audits based on patients' notes. If there is more than one data collector, ask them all to collect data on the same patients and compare their results. An experienced/senior member of the team can also perform a thorough review of the patients as a double-check. This will identify any potential problems before the actual audit takes place.

Data quality

Most national audit organisers will perform checks on data quality. These will often be statistical checks, but may include visits to sites to double-check the data collection. The choice of site is usually based on a random sample, but a site may be chosen if there are particular concerns about data quality there. The purpose of the double-check is to reassure the organisers about the accuracy and integrity of the data returned. This type of check is becoming more common, and should not be seen as a criticism of the local data collection.

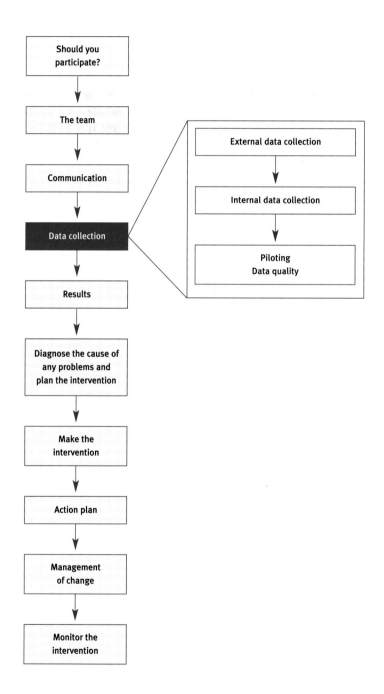

5 Results of the audit

The results of national clinical audits will usually be presented in a way that highlights your local results and compares them with pooled results across the country. Your results may also be compared with a predetermined standard or series of standards. In some national clinical audits, you will have access to your own local results before the pooled results are released.

How representative are your results?

Before looking at your results, you need to consider whether there were any factors that could have affected them or whether anything unusual happened during the data collection period. Ideally, the data should have been collected during a period representative of your 'normal' activity (although, of course, such a 'normal' period rarely exists). If anything could have influenced the results, this has to be borne in mind when interpreting them. Equally, if you are suspicious about the quality of the data, you should double check that they were collected properly.

Ask yourself:
- ► Were you much busier or quieter than usual?
- ► Was there an unusual amount of staff sickness or annual leave?
- ► Did the data collection period coincide with an influenza outbreak that affected your case mix, etc?
- ► Were the data collected properly?

What do your results mean?

It is helpful to consider your results in isolation before comparing them with other centres. This will give you a picture of how you compare against the standards or clinical guidelines on which the audit is based.

There is a temptation to place a lot of emphasis on the rankings given in the tables comparing your results with the national picture. It is one of the strengths of national clinical audits, and the organisers usually give this as one of the reasons why you should take part. However, many factors could potentially affect your placing in the rankings:

- ► A national clinical audit will attract a variety of centres or practitioners from a variety of settings.
- ► The case mix for these centres could be very different.
- ► Some national clinical audits recruit centres in secondary care, tertiary care and primary care.
- ► The results of the national clinical audit are usually presented as anonymised data so you can compare yourself only against an anonymous group of other centres. You will not know which centre is which and whether any are similar to yours. If the organisers present a subgroup analysis comparing similar centres, you may get a better idea of how you performed against those similar centres.

You need to be aware of the limitations of any rankings, while not using this as an excuse for dismissing them.

What should you consider when looking at your local results?

- ► Are some measures more important than others? If so, you need to concentrate on these first.
- ► If a standard has been set, how do your results compare with this standard?
- ► Are there any areas in which you have not performed as well as you would have liked?
- ► Are there any areas in which you performed particularly well? Can you identify any particular strengths in these areas?
- ► Are there any relationships between poor performance in different areas (eg if you performed poorly on three criteria, are these linked in any way)?
- ► Do the qualitative data give any clues about the causes of poor – or good – performance?

How should the comparative data be interpreted?

- ► Are there any unique factors that could affect whether you can directly compare your results with other centres (eg unusual or different case mix, tertiary referral centre, etc)?
- ► Are there any subgroup analyses that will give a better comparison with similar units?
- ► Are you generally above or below the *average*? (Remember that you should be aiming for excellence, not just an average score!)
- ► Are there measures on which you score particularly poorly or highly compared with other units?

▶ Are there some criteria for which the *average* is particularly low? If so, it shows that there is a general problem in many units. Even an above average score here may still indicate poor performance.

▶ Is there anything to be learnt from other units or anything that other units can learn from you (eg have the organisers shared anything about lessons learnt from other units or during the piloting)?

▶ Can you find out why some units do well and how other units have improved their performance?

When you have looked at your results, you will have an idea of whether there are any problems to address, and will also begin to pinpoint the nature of the problems. These issues cannot be dealt with until you have looked at what could be causing them.

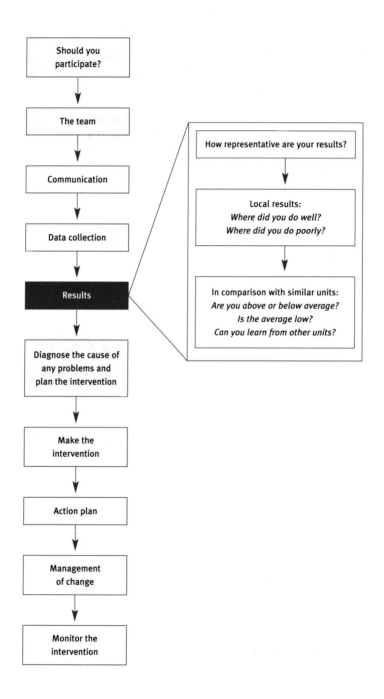

6 Identifying the cause of the problem

People react in different ways when presented with evidence of poor performance from an audit. Some will say that nothing can be changed because:

▶ we need more staff and there's no money for extra staffing
▶ it will take too much work to change it and we don't have the time
▶ the problem is caused by the GPs/consultants/other departments
▶ we have tried already and it didn't work

Others will blame the data, saying:

▶ the data are wrong
▶ the data are not representative

However, you are aiming at a reaction that accepts the problem and wants to deal with it:

▶ this is serious – we must do something about it

Your results may show that you are not performing as well as you had hoped in one or more areas. This suggests there is a problem, but does not necessarily indicate the cause or how to solve it. The results of the national clinical audit can be thought of as identifying a symptom, but a *diagnosis* of the symptom is needed before you can decide on the best treatment.

The job of the local project team is to help develop ways of solving the problems highlighted by the audit.

Diagnosing what is wrong with a patient usually requires the assistance of several members of the healthcare team (eg radiographers for X-rays, pathologists and medical laboratory scientific officers for biopsy results, blood tests, etc). It also requires someone to talk to the patient and listen to what he or she has to say about the symptoms. Diagnosing the cause of poor performance in a clinical team also needs the input of several people, and you will need to listen closely to what the members of the team have to say. Lapses in quality usually have multiple causes and are seldom the fault of one person or department. The solution is rarely simple and will require more than a letter from the senior consultant telling everyone to pull up their socks!

Just as there are tried and tested diagnostic techniques in medicine, so there are techniques that can be used to diagnose problems in the performance of clinical teams (see Appendix 1). Many clinicians shy away from them because they are 'management' techniques and seem unnatural, but they have been used in clinical and non-clinical settings for many years and their usefulness has been proven. If you have not previously used these techniques, it is best to get the assistance of a trained facilitator to help you – talk to your clinical audit department or medical audit advisory group.

All the techniques involve the use of a structured multidisciplinary meeting of all the members of the group affected by the audit. It should be made clear that everyone has a right to speak without criticism, and that the aim of the meeting is not to apportion blame but to solve the problem.

Techniques that may be helpful include:

1 *Brainstorming*: a simple technique to generate ideas on a subject from a group.
2 *Asking 'why' five times*: a way of getting to the true cause of a problem.
3 *Cause and effect diagram*: a way of identifying and analysing multiple causes of a problem.

Types of problems and possible solutions

When thinking about the causes of problems it is worth considering what research demonstrates as the typical causes. These are listed in Table 6.1 (although this list is not comprehensive).[5] Having diagnosed the problem and found the cause(s), you are in a position to decide what action to take. The action should reflect the diagnosis: for example, it is no good organising an educational event if the cause of the problem is inadequate systems.

Your analysis of the situation may have led to specific ideas about what needs to change. Occasionally you will have generated so many ideas for change that it will seem overwhelming – such a big task that the team throws up its hands in horror and gives up! If you or your team has this reaction, it is important to prioritise the work, breaking it up into manageable chunks and conducting it in the right order.

Three simple techniques can be used to help a team prioritise, all of which are useful ways to help a team decide where to start (see Appendix 1):

1 *The nominal group technique*
2 *The Delphi process*
3 *Multivoting*

Table 6.1 Typical causes of problems, the reasons for them and possible solutions[5]

Typical causes	Meaning	Type of action required
Lack of feedback	Practitioners do not have information or possibly do not receive feedback either on how their performance compares with what is expected, or on the consequences of their current performance for patients or other staff	Information – talking ▶ meeting with individuals involved ▶ showing findings ▶ discussing what is needed and why
Lack of knowledge or skill	Practitioners lack the know-how to enable them to perform appropriately	Education ▶ self-assessment exercises ▶ demonstrations ▶ tutoring ▶ reading ▶ formal training ▶ attending clinical meetings
Lack of or inadequate procedures	Practitioners do not perform appropriately because policies, procedures or protocols are not available, accessible, current or user-friendly	Creating or amending procedures
Lack of or inadequate systems	Practitioners do not perform appropriately because performance is impeded by present systems such as: ▶ communications ▶ record keeping ▶ information, etc	Restructuring systems
Lack of motivation	Practitioners are not motivated to perform appropriately due to: ▶ other causes of problems ▶ poor attitudes to work ▶ personal health, emotional, social or other problems	Identifying and addressing individual situations
Lack of or inadequate resources	Practitioners do not perform appropriately because of apparent lack of or inadequate equipment, supplies or staff	Rearranging present resources or establishing priorities for essential new resources

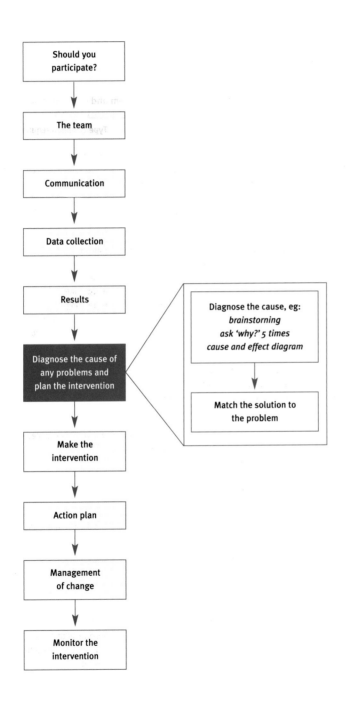

7 Approaches to changing practice

Despite the considerable investment in research relevant to healthcare, there are delays in the implementation of the findings. In many instances this means suboptimal care for patients and unacceptable variation in clinical practice. Many complex factors impede the smooth transition of research findings from publication into everyday practice. Nevertheless, a range of interventions can be used to promote their implementation and change the behaviour of healthcare professionals.

It is generally accepted that simply addressing issues of the dissemination of results is not sufficient to ensure the implementation of findings. Other powerful barriers to developing and, perhaps more importantly, sustaining an evidence-based approach to practice include professional and service culture, and the policy and contractual framework within which services are provided.

Much of the primary research evaluating the effectiveness of interventions in the field of dissemination and implementation are small-scale, and some is methodologically flawed. It has, however, been possible to review the evidence and to provide an indication of which interventions will be effective in improving implementation rates by healthcare professionals.

The passive dissemination of information (eg publication in professional journals, presentation at meetings, mailing of educational material) is generally ineffective, even when the issues being addressed by the research are important and the findings scientifically robust. Despite this, it is perhaps the most widely employed dissemination mechanism used in healthcare, particularly in continuing education.

A number of specific implementation strategies (summarised in Box 3) have been shown to be effective to varying degrees in improving the uptake of research findings.[6]

Changes were shown to occur relatively frequently when barriers to change were addressed or resources deployed to fill any gaps demonstrated in the process. Multifaceted approaches (ie combinations of methods which include two or more approaches) seem to be more

---

Box 3

Interventions to promote behavioural change among health professionals:

Consistently effective interventions

► educational outreach visits
► reminders (manual or computerised)
► multifaceted interventions (a combination including two or more of the following: audit and feedback, reminders, local consensus processes or marketing)
► interactive educational meetings (participation of healthcare providers in workshops that include discussion or practice)

Interventions of variable effectiveness

► audit and feedback (or any summary of clinical performance)
► the use of local opinion leaders (practitioners identified by their colleagues as influential)
► local consensus process (inclusion of participating practitioners in discussions to ensure they agree that the chosen clinical problem is important and the approach to managing the problem appropriate)
► patient-mediated interventions (any intervention aimed at changing the performance of healthcare providers for which specific information was sought from or given to patients)

Interventions that have little or no effect

► educational materials (distribution of recommendations for clinical care, including clinical practice guidelines and electronic publications
► didactic educational meetings (such as lectures)

---

effective than single methods and approaches. This reinforces the fact that you cannot just rely on the feedback of results from a national clinical audit to change practice.

You will need to target your interventions according to the diagnosis of the problem(s) identified. For example, the following may be useful:

► *Educational approaches* (workshops or seminars) when barriers relate to healthcare professionals' knowledge

▶ *Audit and feedback* when healthcare professionals are unaware of suboptimal practice

▶ *Social influence approaches* (local consensus processes, educational outreach, opinion leaders, marketing, etc) when barriers relate to the existing culture, routines and practices of healthcare professionals

▶ *Reminders and patient-mediated interventions* when healthcare professionals have problems processing information within consultations

The presence of organisational barriers may require specific interventions. For example, in East London the development of guidelines on dyspepsia in primary care led to GPs having direct access to testing for *Helicobacter pylori*. Simple interventions such as changing documentation should not be ignored as these may have dramatic effects.[1]

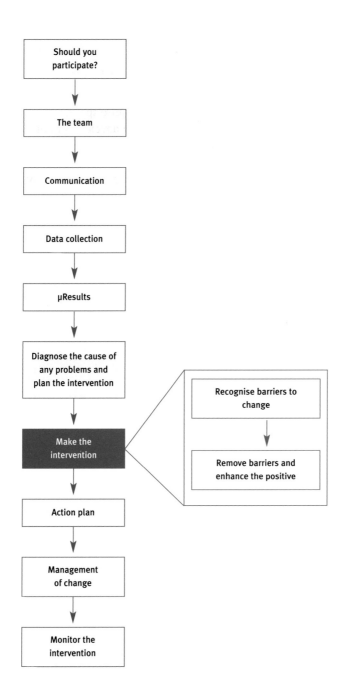

8 Action plan

Having thought about the process of making changes, you will be ready to complete your action plan. (It is a good idea to make a note of the date on which you write the plan.) You will be able to use the plan to work through a series of changes, large and small, and the plan will provide a useful way to check your progress.

By breaking down the tasks/goals into small achievable activities, you can plan all the steps that need to be taken to make the changes which were identified as the most important. It is useful to involve all members of your staff or team in this process, giving each of them an area of responsibility. In this way you can increase involvement, share out the work and, most importantly, share the rewards of success when goals are achieved. Acknowledging others who might be involved is also useful. It can give more junior staff 'permission' to ask for help from more senior staff, and provides a reminder to those who are inclined to 'go it alone'.

Remember that even the smallest task can make a big contribution to achieving change and benefiting patients.

It should be clear how all the tasks relate to the purpose or objectives of the audit. It may be that you have identified a problem that does not obviously connect with the audit objectives because you have had to go back to basics. If so, make a note of this so that you do not lose track of the audit and start following another train of thought.

If resources or further information are needed before the task can be carried out, make a note of this too. It can help you plan your support for the tasks you give to other team members. Identifying resources needed up front should also minimise the stream of reasons why a task has not yet been completed!

Example of action plan documentation

Date written:	Date for review:
Task/Goal	Tick when completed
Purpose (related to objectives)	Person responsible
Others involved	Target date for completion
Resources require	

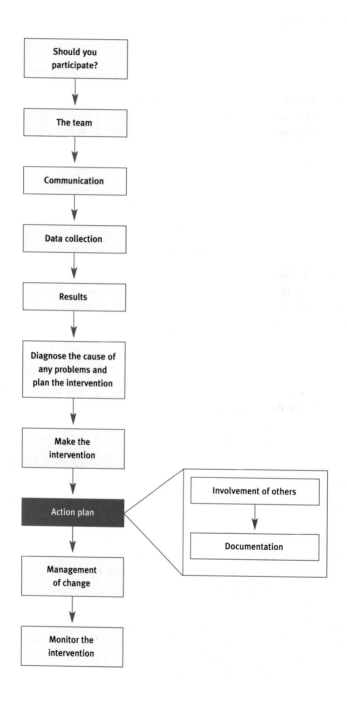

9 Management of change

You have now diagnosed the problem(s), decided on the best approach to changing practice and written an action plan – so you can now sit back and let it happen. **Wrong** – this is when the real work begins!

Achieving and maintaining change which results in improvements in service to patients can be the most frustrating part of the audit process for the team.

Team members often become very involved in the audit process and are highly motivated to achieve improvements. They are lulled into falsely thinking that others will share their enthusiasm for change.

Lasting change does not happen by itself – people backslide and return to their old ways of working. Any change needs management; it is not enough to put on an educational workshop or change the documentation, expecting the problem to go away.

Role of the project manager/project team

Those in charge of the project, whether an individual or a team, must be the leaders of the change process. They should be enthusiastic about the change, and try to lead by example (eg by delivering any parts of the action plan delegated to them).

The project manager/project team has some specific tasks to undertake to ensure that the change runs smoothly:

▶ *Self-education*: find out as much as possible about the change which is to be implemented
▶ *Inform staff*: tell people what is happening and why. By using techniques such as force field (see below and Appendix 1), identify driving and restraining forces in any change taking place. Seek to maximise the driving forces and minimise restraining forces, and also sell the benefits
▶ *Consult staff*: wherever possible, consult staff and involve them in any decisions about change. They will have their own ideas about how to make it work, and will be more committed to the final decision if they have contributed to it

▶ *Organise*: organise the introduction of change. Wherever possible, any change should be piloted to discover and overcome any problems

Reactions to change

Change can be perceived as:

▶ a threat, causing tension and resistance
▶ a questioning of competence
▶ a risk to status
▶ a criticism of what went before

Everyone goes through a series of stages before finally adopting a change as the norm (Table 9.1). You will need to recognise and be aware of what the stages are so that you can help people move on. We all take different amounts of time to pass through each stage. Some people will rapidly move through all of them, while others may appear to get stuck in one phase or even move backwards. Do not try to move individuals on more than one stage at a time (eg from denial to adoption in one go).

Table 9.1 **The stages through which changes are adopted**

Stage	Meaning
Denial	An attempt to deny that the change is necessary or will ever take place
Defence	Defending the *status quo* Protecting the current position
Discard/accept	Resigned to the fact that change will happen and may be necessary Almost a period of mourning
Adapting	Making the new ways work in spite of the problems
Adopt	Accepting the new ways as the norm

Barriers within individuals

Resistance to change is a universal characteristic – it applies to everyone. Understanding the potential barriers will help in developing strategies for change (Box 4).

Box 4

Some general characteristics that affect how easy individuals find it to change:[7]

▶ Willingness to change will vary greatly. Some individuals may be open to new information and positively enjoy taking risks and experimenting. The willingness to adopt change can be categorised as shown in Table 9.2

▶ Younger people usually find accepting change easier than older people

▶ Active membership of a professional organisation will generally indicate a better informed person who is willing to accept innovations

▶ Learning styles will vary, with some people gaining new insights through theory and others by practical experience

▶ Levels of self-confidence will vary from individual to individual

Table 9.2 Ways in which different types of people accept change.

	Early adapters	Majority	Late adapters
Type	Opinion leader	Deliberate, sceptical	Traditional, isolated
Motivation	Intrinsically sees advantage	Social need Peer pressure	Pressure Power
Methods to use	Written methods Scientific arguments Credible sources	Personal sources Opinion leaders Peer activities Reinforcement by social network	Regulations or laws Incentives or sanctions Practical resources

Barriers within groups

No organisation is simply a homogeneous mass of individuals who look and think alike. Rather, there exists within it a number of different groups with different functions to perform. These 'tribes', which develop their own collective identity and 'language', may go under the headings of doctors, nurses, pharmacists, secretarial staff, etc, or be further divided into primary and secondary care. Good quality healthcare requires a number of professions and disciplines to work closely together, but it is easy for a group to split along 'tribal' lines when threatened. Poor results in a national clinical audit can easily lead to one group being blamed for the 'failure'.

Any change that leads to adjustments in the balance of power within a group of people can cause opposition and resentment. If it is decided, for example, that there is a need for a pharmacist on the ward round, this could be seen as moving the pharmacist to a position of greater power within the group. Other members of the group could resent this unless they could see the benefits and were involved in the decision. Changes in perceived status can cause no end of problems – problems often out of proportion to the change itself. Take, for example, moving a consultant to a smaller office or, worse, suggesting two consultants share a secretary! There may be logical reasons for this change that would benefit a lot of people, but it will still be perceived as a threat to the consultants' status and may not be worth the ill feeling that it will cause.

Force field analysis

Force field analysis is a tool that allows you to study a situation that you want to change. It helps you to identify the forces that either aid or hinder the introduction of change by graphically describing the forces that will interact in an attempt to create that change. It is based on the observation that, in general, a situation can be described as a balance between two types of forces:

▶ *driving forces* that help change
▶ *restraining forces* that hinder change

If the driving forces are greater than the restraining forces, change can occur. Once the forces for and against change have been identified, a weighting is given to the forces depending on how strong you think they are. By knowing the pros and cons, you can develop strategies to reduce the impact of the opposing forces and strengthen the supporting forces. You will often find that it is better to try to reduce the hindrances than to increase the driving forces. Remember that no one will like it if you try to force change through. If you find that there are too many restraining forces and too few driving forces, you may have to choose a more realistic goal.

Force field analysis is not an exact science, but can be helpful as a way of making you think about the change you are planning. It can be performed either individually or in a small group.

Selling the benefits

The benefits of changing may be obvious to you and others who have been involved in the audit but, if you want other people to change how they work, you will have to sell the change. First, list the reasons for the change. Think in terms of the benefits for the patients, for the practice/hospital and individuals. The benefits for individuals are probably the most important because few people are so altruistic that they will change what they do solely for the benefit of others. This is not to say that the benefits for patients and the practice/hospital are not important. Healthcare professionals generally have a high degree of concern for others, but this alone may not be enough to persuade people to change their habitual way of working.

Different people can be influenced in different ways. Four different styles can be used to influence people. In practice, each style will appeal to a different type of person. Unless you know your audience well, it will be difficult to predict which style will be most effective and the best way to cope with this is to use a mixture of all four styles in a presentation.

1 *Rewards and punishments*
  This style involves outlining the pluses and minuses of a problem and is characterised by the use of incentives and pressures to control the behaviour of others. It can take the form of offering rewards for compliance and of threatening punishments for non-compliance. It is said to be most effective when it involves a heavier use of praise than criticism (eg if we make the change, we meet the standard, but if we do not change we will be substandard).

2 *Participation and trust*
  The efficacy of this style depends on involving others in the decision-making or problem-solving process. The more others are involved in the decision, the more committed they will become to that decision; this will reduce the amount of follow-up or supervision required. To involve others actively, they should feel that they have something to offer, that their contributions are received and understood by the group and that their efforts are valued. An atmosphere of mutual

trust and co-operation is conducive to participation. You can achieve this by involving them, for example, asking for their opinion and the ways in which they can help.

3 *Common vision*

The common vision is a strategy of articulating a common or shared vision of what the future could be, and of strengthening people's beliefs that the desired outcomes can be achieved through their individual and collective efforts. It involves mobilising the energy and resources of others through appeals to their hopes, values and aspirations. It also activates the feelings of strength and confidence that are generated by being part of a group sharing a common purpose.

Great political leaders such as John F Kennedy and Winston Churchill used this technique to great effect. However, you do not need to be a great charismatic leader to share a common vision. Essentially, you need to be able to share the bigger picture with a degree of enthusiasm and commitment to carry people with you.

4 *Assertive persuasion*

Assertive persuasion uses the power of logic, facts and opinions to persuade others; in other words, for every point you make, you should have the supporting evidence. Evidence-based medicine relies on this type of persuasion to get its points across. The strength of this style is that it appeals to the scientist in the healthcare professional. It is used in most scientific presentations, particularly in audit. However, facts can be disputed and opinions dismissed.

The most persuasive style to use in a presentation to a group is a mixture of all four styles.

Experts suggest that the best order in which to use these styles is:

▶ Common vision
▶ Assertive persuasion
▶ Rewards and punishment
▶ Participation and trust
▶ Common vision

This allows you to set the scene for what you want to achieve and begin to get across the argument for the change from the start. Ending with the vision of how the change will improve the situation helps people take away with them the reason why they have to change. However, the actual order in which the styles are used is not of prime importance. The main point is to use each style, and to begin and end any presentation well.

If you are attempting to persuade an individual, you can pick up clues about which style will be most effective to use. In general, someone who responds to 'rewards and punishment' will tend to look for problems with plans. A 'participation and trust' person will try to get involved with what you are saying. Those who like the 'common vision' approach will get bored with the detail (this will have visible signs!). Finally, the 'assertive persuasion' person will keep asking for examples or want the need for change to be proved.

Experienced negotiators will use these techniques subconsciously; if you watch them, you will be able to see them switch styles. If you are not so experienced, it can be helpful to understand how each style can be used to its best advantage.

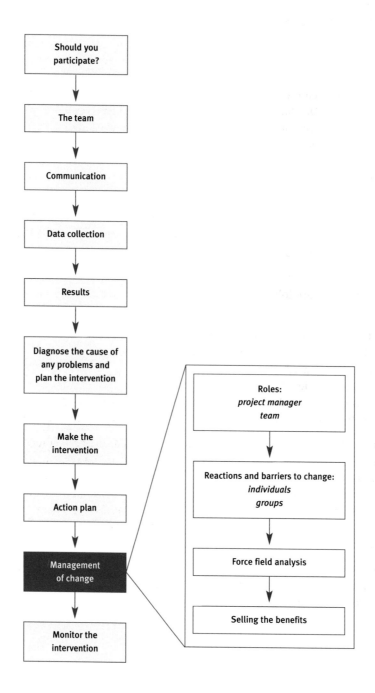

10 Monitoring the action plan

The project team will need to keep a close check on the progress of the action plan. Deadlines can easily slip as other pressures of work take over. If you are not careful, the project can easily get out of control and the impetus be lost. This is not because people deliberately decide not do what they have agreed to do, but because priorities will change. It is the job of the project team to make sure the project keeps on track.

No matter how carefully the team has devised its action plan, something unexpected will go wrong. It is impossible to plan for all eventualities, but if the project is closely monitored you will be able to take remedial action as soon as a problem occurs.

The project leader and project manager need to ensure that all the action points are followed through.

To monitor progress, ask a few simple questions:
- ▶ Has the action plan been implemented?
- ▶ If it could not be implemented, has alternative action been planned or implemented?
- ▶ Are all the deadlines being met?
- ▶ Has the action taken resulted in the goal being achieved?
- ▶ Is there any noticeable difference resulting from the action taken?

After all the action points have been implemented, the project team should confirm that the change has taken place and has had the desired effect. It is not always necessary to repeat the entire audit to check whether or not a change in practice has occurred. The approach to follow-up should reflect the original audit findings. Nancy Dixon suggested a guide to helping teams design an approach to follow-up (Table 10.1).[5]

At the end of this process, you should be able to see that all the effort was worthwhile, and that you have been able to effect real improvements in patient care.

Table 10.1 An approach to a follow-up audit[5]

Audit findings	Follow-up design
A problem revealed by the audit is so critical that it requires immediate action	Establish, immediately and continuously, a way of monitoring the patients or events involved until resolution of the problem is assured
Only a few indicators were not met in the audit	Repeat data collection some time after action has been implemented on only those indicators not met
Widespread variations in findings were revealed	Consider a more detailed audit. For example, if an audit reveals major variations in outcomes, consider doing an audit on aspects of patient care management or process. This may reveal an equivalent amount of variation in processes of care
Many problems involving several indicators were revealed in an audit	Repeat the entire audit some time after actions addressing the problems have all been implemented
Conclusions could not be reached about meeting some indicators because of faulty indicators, definitions, or lack of data	If the indicators measure a critical aspect of patient care, revise the indicators or definitions, or create the data, and repeat the audit
Only a very few variations occurred in the audit on matters which do not have a serious impact on immediate patient care	Note the results, and see if future audits reveal similar occurrences which potentially could suggest a pattern
No problems were revealed as all indicators were met	Reconsider the audit design and indicators, and check if the data were retrieved and presented completely and accurately. If so, ensure that the results are shared positively with all concerned

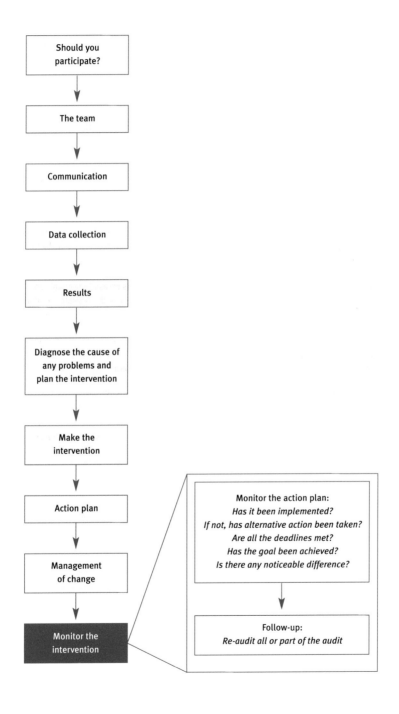

Conclusions

National clinical audits can be a good tool for improving patient care across a number of hospitals and practices. Some national clinical audits are more successful than others, which may be a reflection of how they are organised and implemented. Some teams taking part in a national clinical audit are also more successful than other teams, which is often due to the commitment and skill of the local project team.

In this handbook, we have taken you through how to get the most out of taking part in a national clinical audit. We hope you have been able to make valuable improvements to the way you deliver patient care. If you have, share this with the organisers of the audit and other people in your trust or practice.

Appendix 1
Techniques in more detail[8]

Brainstorming

What it is

A way of collecting the maximum number of ideas on a subject from a group without consideration of the validity or practicality of the ideas.

When to use it

To generate a list of ideas when a group would benefit from having as broad a range of ideas or alternatives as possible.

How to do it

1 Describe the brainstorming process and set the ground rules as follows:
   - There will be no discussion on the practicality or validity of any idea suggested
   - No comments or judgements will be made about any idea, and no joking or whispering
   - There will be no justification discussed for any idea
   - Everyone is encouraged to participate
2 Define the subject of the brainstorm. Try using a question such as 'What are the possible ...?'
3 Give the team a minute or two to think.
4 Ask everybody to call out their ideas.*
5 Write down all ideas on a flip chart. Be sure that every idea is recorded accurately.
6 Decide how the group wants to proceed in discussing the ideas, then proceed with discussing each idea in turn.

Asking 'why?' five times

What it is

A way of getting to the 'true' cause of a problem.

---

* To ensure that everyone participates, ask each person for one idea, and repeat the process until all ideas are recorded. Brainstorming works best among people who know and trust each other, and with a group within which there is little assertion of rank or pecking order. Brainstorming is the basis for other group decision-making techniques.

When to use it

To help a group analyse one potential major cause, identifying what is behind or at the root of the situation.

How to do it

1 Describe the technique and set the ground rules as follows:
   ▶ Only one potential major cause can be analysed at a time. If the team members name other potential causes which they believe are significant, switch to doing a fishbone diagram (see cause and effect diagram)
   ▶ As with brainstorming, all team members' ideas are accepted without judgement
2 Write a problem situation on a flip chart, then ask the team members to name what they think is contributing to the situation. Write down one potential cause.
3 Ask the team members to consider the one potential cause you wrote down and to name what they think is contributing to it. Write down one explanation.
4 Ask the team members to consider the one explanation you wrote down and to name what they think is contributing to the situation contained in the explanation. Continue until the team has answered five times or until they have reached the explanation which they accept is the 'true' one.
5 Begin working on an action plan to address the 'true' cause.

Cause and effect diagram (see opposite)

(also known as fishbone, Ishakawa, tree or fault analysis)

What it is

A way of identifying and analysing multiple causes of a problem.

When to use it

To help a group to structure brainstorming and analysis of potential causes.

How to do it

1 Describe the technique and set the ground rules, which are the same as for brainstorming.
2 Draw a 'fishbone' structure on a flip chart as follows:
   ▶ Fill in the problem, situation, or effect which the team is analysing. Label the spines with potential ways to group or attribute primary causes (eg providers, processes/systems, patients, equipment or other categories).
3 For each of the primary cause spines, ask the team to brainstorm ideas which could be attributed to the primary cause. Secondary causes are drawn as attached to the relevant key spine, and any tertiary causes are attached to the relevant secondary spine.

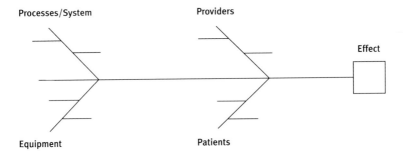

4 When the team has completed brainstorming, ask the members to decide if they want to set priorities among the causes in order to develop an action plan. Then, begin working on an action plan.

The Delphi process

What it is
A structured way to achieve consensus on ideas and establish priorities.

When to use it
To set priorities on ideas using criteria and ratings established by the team.

How to do it
Stage 1 *Generating the ideas*
1 Use brainstorming or stage 1 of the nominal group process to generate the ideas.
2 Be sure all ideas are written down on a flip chart.

Stage 2 *Setting priorities*
1 Decide with the team on the criteria for setting priorities. It is useful to include a time frame in any criteria: for example, the team could say 'important to address in the next three months'.
2 Set a scale with weightings to be used in judging how the criterion applies to each item on the list: for example, for 'importance' the team could use weightings such as 3 for critical, 2 for very important, 1 for important, and 0 for not important.
3 Ask each team member to judge every item on the list in accordance with the agreed criteria and weightings.
4 Record all team members' scores for each item.
5 Calculate the mean of the weighted scores for each item.
6 Place the items in order according to the mean weighted scores.
7 Discuss the next steps for the items with the highest scores.

Nominal group process

What it is

A highly structured way to generate a list of ideas and then to narrow down the list.

When to use it

To generate and process ideas when the team members do not know each other, when some controversy within the group is anticipated, or when a team cannot easily resolve disagreement.

How to do it

Stage 1 *Generating the ideas*

1 Describe the process and set the ground rules, which can be the same as those for brainstorming.
2 Define the subject or question and write it on the flip chart.
3 Ask the team members to write down their ideas in silence, and to work quietly until everyone is finished. Answer any questions for clarification, but do not allow discussion.
4 Ask each person in turn to name one idea from his/her list.*
5 Write down each idea on a flip chart.
6 Continue – quickly – to record all ideas, with the round robin continuing until all ideas are recorded.
7 Make sure everyone understands each idea on the list. If necessary, ask the person who named the idea to clarify it, without discussion. Change the wording of an idea only if its contributor agrees with the proposed change. If two or more ideas appear to be the same, they can be combined if the originators of each idea agree.

Stage 2 *Narrowing down the list*

1 Ask the team members to choose their priorities. If there is a long list, each person may be asked to choose the top three, five or ten, assigning a number from 1 to the number of priorities to be chosen, where 1 equals the lowest priority item.
2 Record all team members' votes for priorities.
3 Identify the ideas voted as top priorities by tallying the ranks assigned to each item and calculating the mean rank for them.
4 Discuss each priority item in turn.

Multivoting

What it is

A way of conducting, with limited discussion and difficulty, a straw poll or vote to select items from a list.

---

* To save time and/or preserve anonymity, the facilitator can collect the lists and then record them together on a flip chart.

When to use it

To identify quickly the ideas on which the team reaches agreement.

How to do it

Stage 1 *Generating the ideas*

1 Use brainstorming or stage 1 of the nominal group process to generate the ideas.
2 Be sure all ideas are written down and numbered on a flip chart.

Stage 2 *Narrowing down the list*

1 Announce the number of votes to be granted to each team member, giving each of them a number of votes equal to one-half the number of items on the list. If the number of items on the list is an odd number, round up to the next even number, then divide by two to derive the number of votes. For example, if there were 12 items on the list, each team member would have 6 votes; if 13 items, seven votes.*
2 Explain that votes may be allocated in any way each team member wishes (eg giving all votes to one item, half the votes to one item and half to another or spread across several items, one vote to several items, etc).
3 Ask each team member to write down his/her votes by first writing the item number or name, then recording the vote.
4 Collect the team members' votes and tally them, preferably on a flipchart.
5 Identify the items with the most votes.
6 Discuss the next steps for the items which have scored highest.

Force field analysis

What it is

A method used to get a view of all the forces for or against a plan so that a decision can be made which takes into account all interests. In effect, this is a specialised method of weighing pros and cons.

When to use it

When a change is planned, force field analysis helps you to analyse all the forces affecting the change and to weigh the pros and cons. By knowing the pros and cons, you can develop strategies to reduce the impact of the opposing forces and strengthen the supporting forces.

How to do it

Stage 1 *Generating the ideas*

1 Start with a well-defined goal or change to be implemented.
2 Draw a force field diagram:
   ▶ Write the goal or change to be implemented on a sheet of paper

---

* If the team is working on an exceptionally long list of items, agree with them a suitable number of votes, such as 10 or 15 for lists of 30 or more items.

▶ Divide the paper into two columns by drawing a line down the middle. Label the left and right columns 'Driving forces' and 'Restraining forces' respectively

3 Brainstorm a list of driving and restraining forces and record them on the chart in the appropriate column. These forces could be people, money, time, external factors, etc – anything that might help or hinder you making a change.

Stage 2 *Scoring the list*

1 Once the driving and restraining forces have been identified, ask the following questions:

▶ Are they valid?

▶ How do we know?

▶ How significant is each of them?

▶ What is their strength?

▶ Which ones can be altered?

▶ Which cannot be altered?

▶ Which forces can be altered quickly?

▶ Which ones can be altered only slowly?

▶ Which forces, if altered, would produce rapid change?

▶ Which forces produce only slow change in the situation?

▶ What skills and/or information are needed and available to alter the forces, and can we get them?

2 Assign a score to each force, from 1 (weak) to 5 (strong). The score is based on (a) the strength of the force and (b) the degree to which it is possible to influence this force.

3 Calculate a total score for each of the two columns.

4 Decide if the goal or change is feasible; if so, devise a manageable course of action which:

▶ weakens restraining forces

▶ strengthens driving forces

▶ creates new driving forces

It is usually better to try to reduce the restraining forces before trying to increase the driving forces. Trying to force change through may cause its own problems as, for example, staff can be annoyed into active opposition to a plan instead of merely not welcoming it.

Bibliography

1 Feder G, Eccles M, Grol R, Griffiths C, Grimshaw J. Using clinical guidelines. *British Medical Journal* 1999; **318**: 728–30.

2 Further information on audit/research design can be found in any good textbook on research methodology or in the following:
   (a) Crombie IK, Davies HTO, Abraham SCS, Florey CduV. *The audit handbook – improving health care through clinical audit.* Chichester: John Wiley & Sons Ltd, 1993.
   (b) Smith R (ed). *Audit in action.* London: *British Medical Journal,* 1992.
   (c) Morrell C, Harvey G. *The clinical audit handbook – improving the quality of health care.* London: Baillière Tindall/Royal College of Nursing, 1999.

3 The Caldicott Committee. *Report on the review of patient-identifiable information.* London: Department of Health, 1997.

4 Dunning M, Abi-Aad G, Gilbert D, Hutton H, Brown C. *Experience, evidence and everyday practice.* London: Kings Fund, 1998.

5 Dixon N. *Medical audit primer.* Romsey: Healthcare Quality Quest, 1991.

6 Bero LA, Grilli R, Grimshaw JM, Harvey E, *et al.* 'Closing the gap between research and practice: an overview of systematic reviews of interventions to promote the implementation of research findings'. *British Medical Journal* 1998; **317**: 465–8.

7 Semple Piggot C, Roe P (eds). *Health gain and how to achieve it.* Uxbridge: Glaxo Pharmaceuticals UK Ltd, 1994.

8 *Getting ahead with clinical audit.* Bristol: NHS Training Directorate, 1994.

Notes